Preparing For Birth: Fathers

Background notes for Pre-natal Classes

Andrea Robertson

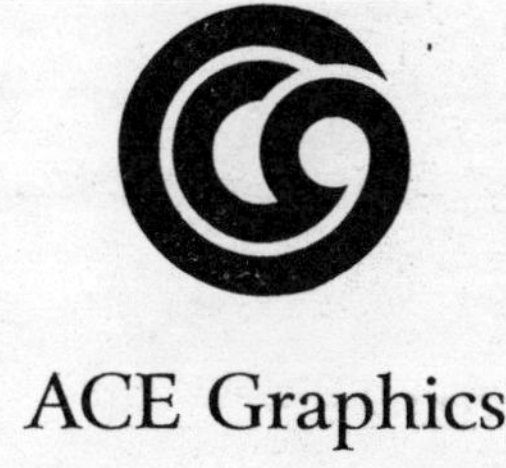

ACE Graphics

Contents

How to use this book

This book is intended to be used in conjunction with its companion volume *Preparing For Birth: Mothers* which contains complementary information, and appropriate cross references will be mentioned throughout this book so that you can easily find the additional information you need.

These books are not intended to offer complete coverage of the topic, since you and your circumstances are very individual. They have therefore been written as "background notes", and if you have further questions, or need additional information, your childbirth educator, midwife or doctor should be able to assist you.

Feedback about the usefulness of this book is always welcome and will help shape future editions. You can contact the author through her publisher at the address given.

Andrea Robertson

So you are going to be a father!

This is an exciting time for both you and your partner. Over the next few months there will be amazing changes in your lives as your family develops. There will be many ups and downs, lots of problems to solve and decisions to be made. You are embarking on a whole new career as a dad, a lifestyle change with enormous benefits and great joy and also heavy responsibilities and concerns. Your whole perspective will change and in the future you will be seeing the world not just through your own eyes, but also those of your children.

It's a wonderful new experience, full of opportunities to develop your strengths and personal skills. You have probably faced major changes to your life before, and the strategies that you used then to weather upheavals will be just as useful now. It is impossible to predict how parenthood will affect you and there is no way of knowing in advance what your baby will be like, what your child will need and how you and your partner will manage the new challenges you will inevitably encounter.

Remember that you already have valuable experience, from being a child yourself, being raised by your own parents and from many important events in your life as you have grown up. These form a solid foundation from which you can develop your own parenting style as a dad. They will also be a resource for you when you are trying to decide how to solve the problems you will encounter with your own children.

You have a very positive and valuable contribution to make to this pregnancy, the birth to come and later with your baby and child. The ideas in this book will help you get started and show you how you can be involved. This pregnancy and birth will never occur again, so make the most of it and enjoy it as much as you can!

KEEPING PREGNANCY AND BIRTH IN PERSPECTIVE

Being pregnant is a natural state for women. Their bodies are cleverly and uniquely designed for childbearing and "having a baby" is not an illness condition that requires medical treatment. Just as your partner is capable of having and enjoying sex, she is capable of creating a baby, giving birth and breastfeeding with the same degree of pleasure and fulfilment. Even though her body is uniquely equipped to produce a baby all by itself, she needs your support and companionship as she discovers her latent talents for motherhood.

Your partner will be undergoing huge changes within her body, many of them seemingly mysterious and some of them challenging. The physiological processes involved in producing a baby are much the same for every woman, yet each woman will respond to these creative urges in her own way. In general, trust her to know what she needs: only she can tell what she is feeling, and the intense personal closeness of her developing baby often enables her to have remarkable insight into the baby's needs as well.

Nature has designed a system for producing babies that is almost always safe and effective. The process has taken thousands of years to perfect and rarely goes wrong, provided that it is left to function as intended and no unnecessary interventions occur. Approximately one woman in ten will develop a complication, either because of her own health or that of the baby, but the remaining nine can produce a healthy baby in a straightforward way.

The medical surveillance techniques that have developed over the years have been designed to help identify and treat the 10% who need this specialised assistance to improve their outcomes, and most of the time these interventions are successful. Sadly, however, some babies and (extremely rarely) women will die, often despite the best efforts having been made. This is "nature's way" of strengthening the species, even though it represents a tragic loss.

YOUR ROLE

The primary role for men over the thousands of years women have been having babies (apart from playing a major part in getting the whole process started!) has been to support and protect the woman during her pregnancy, while the birth is in progress and in the critical early weeks after the birth. To grow a healthy baby a woman needs good food, a calm, safe environment, and freedom from worry or anxiety. These are areas where a nurturing male is especially useful, and by taking on this role, you will be rewarded with a healthy baby and a happy partner, confident in her ability to nurture and raise your child. Much like an insurance policy, plenty of loving support throughout the pregnancy and during birth should result in a better outcome and a significantly reduced chance of problems later on.

So you are going to be a father! CONTINUED

The complexity of the health care system and the many choices on offer need careful consideration. Your partner will need a listening ear and an ally as she explores the kind of care available from the various health professionals and as she chooses an appropriate place to give birth. Working together to make the necessary decisions will make these tasks easier and more rewarding.

You bring a unique perspective to these decisions: you are closely involved, yet because you are not the one actually giving birth you may find it easier to see the bigger picture. It can also be a difficult position, since your emotional involvement can tend to cloud your view, and there will be times when you need to put your partner's views before you own.

YOUR NEEDS

Becoming a father can be an emotional and physically draining time. Many men report similar ups and downs as their partners during the pregnancy, sometimes felt as see-sawing emotions and at other times as physical symptoms.

Every father has been down this road before you, and all have fascinating stories to tell of their experiences. It can be enormously helpful to talk to other men about their reactions, and you'll discover that these feelings are remarkably common. If you are concerned, seek appropriate help, so that you can relax into your new lifestyle with confidence.

There is nothing to stop you accompanying your partner on her pre-natal visits to her caregiver. Going together gives you an opportunity to discuss your own needs, and to have your questions answered. A competent caregiver should be very willing to make time for you too and recognise your rights as well.

Above all, take the time to participate and enjoy these new experiences. Don't be afraid to ask questions or to seek help from those around you. You'll be surprised at how willing people are to offer suggestions!

Choosing the best maternity care for your family

You and your partner have a variety of health care options to consider for pregnancy care and these are described below. Not all of these services are available in all communities and a first step might be to take some time to investigate what is on offer locally and further afield. The earlier you start in the pregnancy the more time you will have time to evaluate the services available. Don't hurry these decisions. Weighing up the options and speaking to the relevant people will ultimately help you feel more comfortable about the decisions you've made. You always have the right to a second opinion and to change caregivers at any time.

PROFESSIONAL CAREGIVERS

Many parents give little thought to choosing a midwife or doctor and rely on recommendations from friends or their family doctor. However, choosing a caregiver to assist your partner is the most important decision that you will make.

There is clear research evidence that the major influences on the outcome of the birth (that is, the health of mother and baby) are the attitudes, practices and philosophy of the primary caregiver. The way this person views birth, their management style and their level of commitment to the normal birth process will determine how they care for your partner and the services they perform.

It is worthwhile discussing your goals for the birth with your partner and then working together to seek the caregiver who will best assist you achieve this outcome. It is quite acceptable to "shop around" for appropriate health care and interviewing potential caregivers can be rewarding. A list of questions that could be asked is included at the end of this section. To find the names of health professionals who offer pregnancy and birth services in your area, you could contact the local hospital, the community health centre, women's health clinic, or baby health centre.

The midwife

The World Health Organisation recommends that midwives should be regarded as the best caregivers for normal, healthy pregnant women, and indeed, round the world, most babies are born with the assistance of a midwife, either in a hospital or at home.

A midwife has training in the management of normal pregnancy, birth and newborn care. She (there are a few male midwives, but most are female) can recognise any problems that arise and will refer to specialists as necessary. They have wide experience of normal birth and offer a range of non-medical techniques for promoting safe outcomes and for dealing with the pain of labour. Midwives have a separate training from nurses and are recognised, not as "obstetric nurses" but as practitioners in their own right.

All maternity hospitals are fully staffed with midwives. If you are a public patient, or using standard health care services for the pregnancy and birth, your partner will see a midwife for her pre-natal check-ups and have a midwife to assist at the birth and also post-natally. There may be no choice in who she sees, although some hospitals offer special clinics staffed by midwives alone, or a team midwifery program where a small permanent team of midwives care for a designated group of women. You can enquire about these services at the hospital. Hospital based midwifery services are usually free.

In some areas, independent midwifery is available, either on a private (fee paying) basis, or as an outreach program from the local hospital. An independent midwife will provide all the care during pregnancy, labour, birth and in the first weeks after the birth. She may work on her own or with a partner to provide back up. Independent midwives usually offer homebirth but in some locations they have visiting rights at the local hospital and can assist at births in that setting.

Midwives in private practice charge a range of fees according to their services. Should it become necessary, the midwife can refer to a doctor (probably an obstetrician) for specialised tests or to manage complications if they arise. You may have to pay additional fees for these medical services. Be sure to ask about the costs involved for all these services in advance, and to check whether they are covered by any medical insurance that you may have.

The General Practitioner

In some communities General Practitioners (GPs) offer maternity care. Although not as comprehensively trained as obstetricians, they usually have additional qualifications in obstetrics and often undertake Caesarean sections, especially in rural areas where no obstetrician is available. Sometimes, a GP may "share care" with a midwife, alternating visits or just seeing the woman once or twice during the pregnancy. In other locations they provide the pre-natal care for hospital patients who will eventually give birth in the local hospital assisted by either the midwife on duty or by themselves.

Choosing the best maternity care for your family CONTINUED

Because you may already know them, and as they will usually care for your family following the birth, seeing your GP throughout your pregnancy offers the advantage of continuity of care over a longer period of time.

GP services are usually free as part of the public health system, but in some places, an additional fee may be charged, especially where patients have private health insurance. It would be wise to check this in advance.

The obstetrician

The obstetrician is specially trained in the management of complicated pregnancies and births. Any client that a midwife considers "high risk" would normally be referred to an obstetrician who would take over the case and assist the woman to give birth in an appropriate hospital setting. If a woman has an existing health condition, such as diabetes or high blood pressure, other specialists may be consulted. Additional fees will be payable for these specialised services, however most of these costs should be covered by the public health system or by private health insurance.

Some expectant parents choose to engage an obstetrician even for a birth which they expect will be normal and uncomplicated, in case a problem develops later that requires specialised assistance. The statistics show however, that this approach leads to higher rates of interventions in birth such as Caesarean section and forceps. The reasons for this are unclear however a likely cause is that many obstetricians follow the medical model, which anticipates problems rather than managing birth as a natural process. Unnecessary intervention in birth adds considerably to the costs of maternity services for the community as a whole and to individual parents in particular, and ultimately may not result in a better birth outcome.

Questions to ask when choosing a professional care giver for birth:

Many pre-natal visits to caregivers leave little time for discussion. To give you the time you will need, you could try booking the last appointment of the day, when there is usually more time available. When you have many questions to ask, going together will encourage the caregiver to spend more time answering your questions.

To help you decide if this is the right person to assist you with the birth, here are some issues worth raising:

- What services do you offer for the pregnancy, labour and birth and after the baby is born?
- What pattern of visits do you suggest?
- Are you in a solo practice or a partnership? Who are your partner(s) and do you all have the same approach to the way you practice? Can an appointment be made to meet the partner?
- Are you available at all times, even weekends, or do you have other arrangements in place for weekends and evenings?
- Do you have holidays planned for when the baby is due, and who will cover for you if you are away?
- What are your charges for pregnancy care, labour and birth and postpartum follow up? How much of this fee is covered by the public health system and what must I pay from my own pocket, or from my private health insurance?
- If an anaesthetic becomes necessary for either pain relief during labour or a Caesarean section, which anaesthetist do you usually call?
- If the baby requires paediatric follow up, whom do you recommend for this service?
- What pregnancy tests do you suggest we consider? What are the advantages and disadvantages of the tests for the woman and the unborn baby? Will you be comfortable if we choose not to have a particular test, or want to try an alternative approach?
- What are your preferences for labour management, including drugs for pain and positions for birth? Have you ever assisted a woman giving birth in a squatting or kneeling position on a floor mat?
- How often do you perform an episiotomy? How often do you use forceps? (More information on these procedures can be found in *Preparing For Birth: Mothers*).
- Will you be comfortable if we choose to have additional support people present?
- What preparation do you recommend? Where can I attend pre-natal classes?

Give yourself time to consider the answers you receive and to talk them over with your partner. Remember that if your initial choice of caregiver proves unsatisfactory, you can change to another at any time during the pregnancy, providing that the new caregiver is available and willing to assist.

CHOOSING A BIRTH PLACE

The environment in which a woman labours and gives birth has a major effect on the birth. Your partner's physiological responses will be affected by her surroundings and the result can either speed or delay the process. Her main need is to feel safe and protected from danger or harm, since during the hours of labour she will feel particularly vulnerable.

Many expectant parents assume that their baby will need to be born in a hospital. The World Health Organisation states that normal, healthy pregnant women may wish to consider a number of options, and that for these women, giving birth in their own home is the safest option. In choosing a place to give birth, the availability of suitable caregivers to assist you will be a major factor. You may find that some birth places are impractical because there is no caregiver able to provide the necessary service in that location.

Be prepared to support your partner's choice. She may want to arrange several alternatives and make her final decision during labour. For example, she may make a booking at the hospital, but choose a midwife who can assist her in either your home or at the hospital, depending on how the labour develops and how she feels at the time.

Home birth

The availability of home birth depends largely on the availability of midwives who provide this service. In some places, home birth is provided through the local health authority, and in other areas engaging the services of an independent midwife will be necessary. Doctors rarely provide home birth services, since they are primarily required to manage problems in appropriate hospital settings.

You may need to make extensive enquiries to determine the availability of home birth where you live. You can ask at your local hospital, community health centre, women's health centre, Family Planning Agency or check the telephone book for listings of midwives and home birth support groups.

Advantages

- Freedom to "do your own thing" in the privacy of your own home.
- No need to make special arrangements for other children.
- Your partner will be naturally in charge, since this is her own place.
- You may invite anyone you wish to attend and participate.
- Reduced risk of medical technology or drugs being used routinely – you will be asked to consent to every procedure.
- Reduced risk of infection.
- The baby will be welcomed into its own home and family with little chance of separation or disruption.
- No need for you to make hospital visits to see the baby – the midwife will provide post natal care in your home.

Disadvantages

- Your home must have basic equipment – telephone, plenty of hot water, ready access, and should be within 20 minutes of the nearest hospital.
- If there is a complication with the labour, your partner will need to transfer to the hospital, which can be traumatic.
- Although the midwife will carry basic medical equipment for most situations, if there is a problem with the baby, emergency transfer to the nearest hospital may be necessary.
- You will need to arrange for additional help in the home following the birth, as your partner will still need to rest with the baby for the first days, even weeks.

Hospital labour ward

The majority of women give birth in a standard hospital labour ward. Care in the hospital is usually free, however, if you have private insurance you may be asked to pay, particularly if you elect to use better facilities, such as private rooms, reserved for those who can pay the extra fees.

Labour wards vary in their facilities and the degree of privacy they offer, and a visit during the pregnancy will help you to decide if this is where you want to be for the birth. Prepare for this visit by reading the appropriate sections in *Preparing For Birth: Mothers* to gain the necessary background information. During this visit, you may wish to raise the following issues:

- Are there any restrictions on whom we can invite to the birth?
- What are the hospital policies regarding:
  - Position for labour and birth? Is giving birth on a floor mat acceptable, if requested?
  - Procedures that are routinely performed, unless specifically refused?
- What equipment do you have to enable women to get comfortable during labour: extra pillows, armless chairs, floor mats, bean bags, hot packs?
- Do you have showers or baths available for use during labour to ease the pain?
- Breastfeeding – is the hospital accredited as being "Baby Friendly" using the World Health Organisation's guidelines?
- What are the hospital's rates for Caesarean section, forceps, epidurals, episiotomy and induction?
- What costs will be involved in using the hospital? Can I pay for additional services?

- What facilities do you have for the support people?
- Where do I park the car?
- When do you suggest we come to the hospital in labour?

Birth Centres

Some hospitals have additional facilities, called Birth Centres, that are designed to be as home-like as possible. These units are usually set up as a separate unit, and have their own staff of midwives to oversee the pre-natal care and the birth. They aim to enable women to give birth with as little intervention as possible, however, should the woman require medical assistance or the use of pain relieving drugs, she can be transferred to the labour ward, which is usually nearby.

Since a Birth Centre operates as a separate facility within the hospital it is important to register for their program as early as possible. They are very popular and often set strict limits on the numbers of clients that they can take. As they are part of the regular hospital services there is usually no charge made for care in a Birth Centre.

In some places, free standing Birth Centres have been established to provide home-like births for those who wish to pay for a private service. These units are usually staffed by independent midwives, who have back up arrangements with local obstetricians and hospitals. Ask for full details of the services they offer and the costs involved.

EXTRA SUPPORT PEOPLE

During labour and birth, having an extra helper to assist you can make it much easier to provide your partner with the support she needs. A spare pair of hands to massage, hold and comfort her can be very welcome, as it enables you to take a break from time to time to re-energise, and to share the practical tasks and responsibilities. The presence of supportive birth companions has been shown to reduce a woman's need for painkilling drugs in labour and to make her labour shorter.

Think carefully about whom you could invite to fulfil this role – your partner should be the one to issue the invitation, and you need to be comfortable working with the extra person as well. Some women like to choose a close friend or relative, perhaps their mother or sister. Other parents seek the help of their childbirth educator. It is not necessary for support people to have given birth themselves, although having people around who had positive birth experiences can be reassuring. There are practical considerations as well:

- Will the helper be available – can they get time off work if necessary, or arrange babysitting quickly for their own children?
- What is their attitude to birth? Do they see it as a normal, natural event or are they full of anxieties and fear, perhaps stemming from their own experiences?
- Do you and your partner feel very comfortable with this person? Women sometimes want to be naked, and to use the toilet or vomit, and it is important that these necessary behaviours are not seen as offensive or alarming by birth companions.
- Would you feel comfortable asking this person to leave, if you felt it was not working out well?
- Are they prepared to really help and support, not just to be a witness? Would they be willing to attend pre-natal classes to learn useful comfort techniques for the labour?

It is helpful to spend some time with the extra support people during the pregnancy to discuss everyone's role and the practical assistance they can offer. Being a birth companion is a statement of commitment to a woman and her family – a real honour and privilege, and this should be understood by everyone concerned. It should not be seen as a service, for which payment is required.

PRE-NATAL CLASSES

Good quality pre-natal classes can help you feel well equipped with practical skills for use during labour, pregnancy and the post-partum period. Most parents would expect to attend some kind of educational sessions, and a variety of programs are available. Look for a program that involves you both and which also welcomes your extra support people. Shopping around is also recommended, as some programs may be more suitable for your needs than others.

Points to look for in a pre-natal class program:

- At what point in the pregnancy are they scheduled? Early pregnancy sessions give you a chance to get vital information on birth place and care givers when you are making the initial decisions.
- Parenting classes in the middle of the pregnancy will address issues that are important at that time, such as making lifestyle changes and getting ready for the baby. Sessions on birth are best left till the end of the pregnancy so that the information and practical skills are fresh in your mind for the big event. There are many variations on these formats!

Choosing the best maternity care for your family CONTINUED

- How large are the class groups? In many areas, preparation for parenthood programs are popular, resulting in large group sizes. Smaller, more intimate groups of 6–8 couples are more effective in meeting your needs, and can offer a more individual approach.
- Who leads the program – a single educator or a team? A single educator for the whole series is usually better from an educational viewpoint and also offers continuity. A team, however, may enable you to meet various people whom you may wish to consult later, such as the Maternal Child Health Nurse, or the Nursing Mothers Association representative.
- What is covered by the program? Ask about the topics included and the philosophy – are you encouraged to develop your own approach to birth, to rely on your own skills and resources, or are you being readied to accept what the hospital is prepared to offer?
- Are other resources available if you need them, such as a lending library, background research information, phone numbers of useful support agencies and an after hours number for the educator if you have a question?

Your childbirth educator will be better able to help if you let her know your concerns. As a resource person, she will know where to get any extra information or assistance you might need. Many have additional qualifications, such as being a midwife, and ideally should have completed special training in education.

To find the pre-natal programs in your area, you can ask your caregiver or at the hospital. Independent, community based educators may be listed in the telephone book, or through other community services, such as women's health services or Family Planning Clinics. In some communities, organisations dedicated to childbirth education and related services have been set up, often on a voluntary "parent-to-parent" basis. They provide easy access to the network of parents in your area, and contact numbers for them can usually be found in the telephone book.

Strategies for increasing safety and security during labour and birth

No matter where or with whom your partner chooses to give birth, there are some things you can do to increase her sense of safety and security. The main strategy is to increase her privacy, through:

- Reducing the number of people in the room.
- Taking her to another room away from people (bathroom, toilet).
- Giving her time on her own, but stay nearby, perhaps outside.
- Making the room darker: dimming the lights, closing the curtains, drawing the blinds.
- Lowering the noise level: remaining quiet, not talking; staying still and avoiding walking around.
- Turning down the monitoring machine.
- Positioning her facing a wall or corner, not the door.
- Covering her with a sheet or blanket to create a "cocoon".
- Maintaining calm surroundings – get help yourself if you are anxious.
- Consulting the midwife if you are unsure of what is happening.

All of these simple measures will enhance her normal physiological responses during labour. You can establish these conditions for her and this will be a significant contribution to her labouring comfortably and safely.

Being prepared...

During the last weeks of the pregnancy, spending some time preparing for the coming events will avoid rushes and help you to feel confident and ready. As you await the arrival of you baby there are a number of things you can do:

Visit your partner's midwife or doctor if you haven't done so already, so you can make their acquaintance. This would also be a good time to discuss any issues you have about the birth, and to support your partner in negotiating any special requests she may have.

Assemble your "goody bag" for labour. There is a list of useful items in *Preparing For Birth: Mothers*. Add anything that you feel will make the time in labour more comfortable for you and your partner.

Prepare some snacks for labour, such as sandwiches (keep them in the freezer until you need them), drinks, packets of fruit and nut mix, high energy food bars and blocks of chocolate.

If you have an off-peak electricity hot water service, arrange to have it temporarily switched over to "continuous heat", so that there is a plentiful supply of hot water during the early stages of labour while she is at home.

Make arrangements for babysitters for your other child(ren) and perhaps pets during labour. You may want to have someone close by who can come quickly to your house, for example, in the middle of the night, rather than having to take the child(ren) to them.

Prepare a number of meals and store in the freezer for use after the baby is born. Cook extra portions of meals during the last few weeks and make left overs into meals that can be defrosted later when time is precious, and food is essential. Meals that will not spoil if there is a sudden need to attend to the baby are useful, and foods that re-heat quickly are also handy.

Keep the car topped up with petrol – you don't want to stop for petrol on the way to the hospital.

Make a dry run to the hospital so you can find it easily. Check out the parking and locate the entrances that are used during the day and at night.

Put some clean, old towels inside a plastic bag and store in the car, in case the unexpected occurs on the way to the hospital (waters breaking, the baby being born!). A plastic container with a tight fitting lid, such as an ice-cream container, would also be useful, in case she feels sick, or you need something to hold the placenta.

Make a sign for the front door, such as "We are attending to the baby right now and can't come to the door. Please call back later or phone______ ", or "New parents catching up on sleep – please don't disturb!".

Record a new message for the answering machine that can be played during pregnancy ("no, the baby hasn't yet arrived, but we will call you when it does...") and afterwards ("we are attending to the baby right now and cannot take your call....")

Arrange to take time off work to be with your family after the baby is born. If you need someone to cover for you on an emergency basis, make these arrangements well in advance.

Obtain copies of the birth registration forms and any other forms that may be applicable, such as Family Assistance forms, from the appropriate government agency.

Check there is film in your camera, for those first pictures of the new baby. If you are planning to take photos during the birth, choose high speed film that will operate in low light conditions. This will avoid having to use a flash, which can be very distracting.

Prepare a list of family and friends to notify of the baby's arrival. Be ready to organise the visiting so that your partner is not constantly bombarded with well-meaning guests who need entertaining. One way to do this is to arrange a "baby welcoming party" when everyone comes at the same time. This may be less tiring and easier on the household, especially if you take charge of the arrangements and catering.

Discuss new arrangements for household chores with your partner. She will be fully occupied with the baby most of the time, and will need to share basic tasks such as shopping, cooking and cleaning. Decide what chores are essential and plan how these will be done. You will need to make time on weekends to do some of these things, and be ready to contribute daily as well. Look for time-saving short cuts (such as pre-prepared nutritious meals, nappy wash services, clothes dryers) and be prepared to lower your standards for the household in the short to medium term.

Plan some special events for the two of you in the days around the baby's guesstimated birth day. Intimate dinners for two, going to a movie, visiting close friends, picnics and visits to art galleries etc are all things you will have to put on hold for some time after the baby arrives. Having a special event to enjoy also makes the tedious waiting more bearable, especially if the baby decides to come a little later than was expected.

Troubleshooting

Pregnancy and birth are healthy conditions for most women. Left alone, nature has designed a process that will usually produce a baby in peak condition and a mother primed to nurture and protect her baby.

Your partner will be offered many tests, drugs and obstetric interventions during her pregnancy and labour. She should be given full information about the risks and benefits associated with these, plus time and support to enable her to make considered decisions. She will look to you for assistance and guidance and you may be asked to help her choose appropriately. During labour, when she is unable to participate fully in the decision-making process because she is concentrating on the labour itself, she may rely on you to convey her wishes to the staff.

Sometimes health carers want to intervene during pregnancy or birth and take control of what is happening. They may believe that by managing labour actively, potential problems may be avoided. The research assembled by the World Health Organisation shows that for at least 80% of women the birth process needs no intervention and that treating it as a medical condition may cause rather than prevent problems.

When your partner is being offered tests during her pregnancy or drugs and obstetric interventions during labour, remember to ask the following basic questions:

1. What is the test/drug/procedure being offered?
2. Why do you think it is necessary right now?
3. How will it be carried out/given/done?
4. What effects (positive and negative) will it have on the mother?
5. What effects (positive and negative) will it have on the baby?
6. What are the alternatives?
7. How will this test/drug/procedure alter the treatment of the woman/the baby?
8. What will happen if we do nothing?

There are many things you can do to help and support her when conditions change during pregnancy and birth, and especially if complications do arise. Even in a straightforward birth, there will be times when your practical assistance is invaluable, and your contributions will make a significant impact upon her well being.

The list below describes some of the situations you may encounter, and offers some practical solutions you can consider. *Italics* indicates additional entries – check these for further ideas. When trying the suggestions remember:

- All women are different and each of their labours is unique. What works for one woman or one labour may not be useful another time.
- Think creatively about the options. Regard each situation as a problem with a number of different possible solutions.
- Allow time, and if one solution doesn't work, don't be concerned about making changes – try another idea. After all, it is not possible to make correct decisions all the time!

Trouble Shooting – Problems in pregnancy

The membranes break and there are no contractions

Signs:
A sudden gush of fluid – between half and two cups of fluid. Nothing else happens.

Possible reasons:

- The labour will be starting soon, probably within the next 48 hours.
- The baby is positioned with its spine against your partner's spine, and this places an uneven pressure on the membranes containing the amniotic fluid, making them more likely to break early.

Remedies:
Check for these positive signs , which you can discuss with the midwife over the phone:

- the escaping fluid is clear or flecked with white (she can collect this fluid on a sanitary pad),
- the baby is settled well down in the pelvis (engaged) often – indicated by her frequent need to use the toilet over the past days or weeks,
- she is about 40 weeks pregnant,
- the baby can be felt moving inside and
- she cannot feel any loops of umbilical cord in her vagina.

If she is earlier than 37 weeks, take her to the hospital as soon as you can, as the baby may be born prematurely.

If she can feel the *umbilical cord in her vagina*, take her to the hospital immediately.

If the *fluid is coloured* (it can vary from pale yellow to dark green) alert the hospital by phone and take your partner in to be checked by the midwife. If all is well, you may either come home again to await the start of contractions or stay nearby. Avoid staying in the labour ward if there are no contractions, since it is likely that a set time limit will be applied, after which there will be pressure to start the labour artificially *(induction)*.

Carry on with your usual routines, especially eating and sleeping at normal times. Include a supper snack before bed.

Make sure that nothing (tampons, fingers, speculum etc) enters her vagina. The escaping fluid will keep the area sterile and make infection very unlikely.

Maintain your own energy by regularly eating and resting too. When it begins, the labour may be slow, and you may miss sleep later.

Bleeding in pregnancy: bright, fresh blood

Signs:
Fresh, bright blood trickles out of the vagina.

Possible reason:

- Fresh, bright bleeding indicates an emergency, and usually means that the placenta has become partly detached from the wall of the uterus.
- Bright bleeding can also occur during the last weeks of pregnancy if the placenta is partly covering the cervix. Once the cervix begins to soften and open, bleeding occurs where the placenta becomes detached from the opening cervix.

Remedies:
If there is fresh bleeding, take your partner to the hospital immediately. Telephone first to alert them to your arrival, and take her prepared bag, as she will probably be admitted to hospital for observation.

Trouble Shooting – Problems in pregnancy CONTINUED

Bleeding in pregnancy: spots of blood	**Signs:** Small spots of blood appear, sometimes with a mucous discharge. **Possible reason:** • Spots of blood can occur after sexual intercourse or after an internal examination by the doctor or midwife if the tiny blood vessels around the cervix are damaged. • Spotting, especially when accompanied by a mucous discharge, may be a signal that the cervix is getting ready for labour. **Remedies:** If you have had recent sexual intercourse, spots of blood may appear. They will disappear as the broken blood vessels in the cervix heal. If there are spots of blood in a mucous discharge, then wait for further signs of labour to develop. These may take days or even weeks to appear. Carry on with normal daily activities while you wait, especially eating and sleeping at the usual times. If you have any doubts about what you are seeing, telephone the hospital and speak to a midwife regarding your concerns. Encourage her to rest and conserve her strength. Avoid long tiring walks, strenuous household activities and other forms of exercise. Keep her calm and unworried. Labour will start when her body and baby are ready.
The baby is lying in an unfavourable position for labour and birth	**Signs:** The midwife has reported that the baby is not well positioned for an easy birth. **Reasons:** • It is not always possible to know why some babies adopt awkward positions. It may be due to the shape of your partner's pelvis, the size of the baby or a combination of these factors. • The location of the placenta may be preventing the baby from turning head down. **Remedies:** During pregnancy, the midwife or doctor may be able to turn the baby using massage. See *breech birth* for a fuller description of this technique. Acupuncture may be successful in getting the baby to turn. You will need to find a qualified acupuncturist to assist you with this. Moxa sticks (see *breech birth*) may also be tried. During labour, the baby may be encouraged to turn by adopting forward leaning position, supported by a chair, bean bag or cushions. Pelvic rocking in this position can also help "jiggle" the baby around. This can be started in the pregnancy and continued right through labour. If the baby remains lying across the abdomen a *Caesarean section* will be necessary.
The baby is in a breech position	**Signs:** The midwife or doctor can feel the baby's head at the top of the uterus. Your partner may also be able to feel the hard round head high under her ribcage. An ultrasound may have confirmed your caregiver's suspicions. **Possible reasons:** • No-one can be sure why some babies decide to adopt this position however it may be due to the location of the placenta or the size and shape of her pelvis in comparison to the baby. • It may be the baby's preference to be "head up" rather than "head down". **see Remedies over**

Trouble Shooting – Problems in pregnancy CONTINUED

The baby is in a breech position	**Remedies:** Most babies will turn before the end of the pregnancy, and only about 3% are actually born breech. To encourage the baby to turn during the pregnancy, a number of remedies can be tried, and these are described in *Preparing For Birth: Mothers*. Although a *Caesarean section* is often suggested, research indicates that breech babies can be born safely through the vagina. An upright position where the pelvis can open freely to its maximum capacity will reduce the risk of pressure on the baby's head as it is being born. Leaning forward either standing or kneeling, supported on the bed, a chair or against you will give the doctor or midwife maximum room to assist whilst ensuring that the pelvis can open easily. Discuss this option with your caregiver in advance so they are prepared to assist. Avoid an epidural which will restrict mobility, and make it harder to adopt an appropriate position.
The umbilical cord appears in the vagina or between her legs	**Signs:** Loops of the cord can either be felt or even seen. **Possible reason:** • This is a rare event. Sometimes when the membranes break the gush of fluid released from around the baby sweeps the cord along and it becomes trapped between the baby's head and the cervix. • This is is more likely to occur of the baby is not snugly fitted into the lower part of the uterus, for example if the baby is in a *breech position*. **Remedies:** Get her to the hospital as fast as you can by ambulance or in your own car, having telephoned first to alert the midwife of your predicament. If the cord is hanging down between her legs, wash your hands, then gently push it just up inside her vagina. Place a pad in her knickers to keep the cord inside. Make her kneel on the back seat of the car, with her head and chest on the seat and her bottom high in the air. This will help keep the weight of the baby off the cervix and reduce the pressure on the cord. Cover her to keep her warm. When you arrive at the hospital, she will probably be taken to theatre for an immediate *Caesarean section*.
The pregnancy has extended beyond the anticipated date of the birth	**Signs:** The due date has passed and there are no signs that labour is about to begin. **Possible reasons:** • The estimated due date is incorrect. • The baby is not yet ready to be born. • Your partner is not yet ready to give birth – perhaps she needs more time to prepare either physically or emotionally. **Remedies:** Recalculate the due date in consultation with the midwife. Use the self-help suggestions listed under induction to try and start the labour. Be patient – as long as your partner and the baby are well it is best to wait for labour to begin naturally.

Trouble Shooting – Problems in labour

When do I take her to the hospital?

Signs:
Feeling anxious about when you should go the hospital.
Feeling pressured to take her to the hospital.

Possible reasons:

- You may be unsure about what is happening and need reassurance or information.
- You may have been advised to come to hospital when certain symptoms appear, such as the waters breaking.

Remedies:
Phone the labour ward and speak to the midwife. She can offer useful suggestions and guidance about when to go to the hospital.

Consult your partner, and be guided by her feelings. Labouring women are usually the best judges of when they need to be in their chosen birth place.

Get everything ready well in advance so there are no last minute rushes:

- put her bag in the car (and lock it)
- prepare the house for your departure
- make any necessary arrangements regarding pets
- notify your workplace
- call your chosen support person(s)

and then either assist your partner or give her some space to get used to the labour (she will tell you what she needs right now).

It is not always wise to notify your relatives that the labour has started. They often become anxious, wanting to know what is happening and telephone frequently (either your home or the hospital) to seek progress reports. This added pressure may interfere with her ability to labour effectively.

Unplanned homebirth, or birth on the way to the hospital

Signs:
The labour is progressing very quickly.
Your partner has an sudden uncontrollable urge to push while still at home, or on the way to the hospital.
Your partner can feel the baby's head in her vagina.
You can see the baby's head.

Possible reasons:

- A very quick and easy labour!
- The baby doesn't want to wait.
- Usually a second or subsequent baby.

Remedies:
Remember that a labour proceeding this smoothly is usually safe for both mother and baby.

If you are within 5–10 minutes of the hospital, decide if you can get there in time. You could call an ambulance or drive her yourself. If using your own car, have her assume an "all fours" position on the back seat of the car, to slow contractions a little. Take some clean bath towels and a plastic container (with a lid) or a plastic carry bag.

If she suddenly has to give birth while you are driving to the hospital, turn off the road, and try and find a quiet place away from traffic. Avoid dangerous dashes to the hospital at high speed. Follow the instructions over.

continued over

Trouble Shooting – Problems in labour CONTINUED

Unplanned homebirth, or birth on the way to the hospital (continued)	Prepare for the imminent arrival of the baby: • Telephone for assistance if there is time: the ambulance service or the labour ward at the hospital. • Encourage her to go into the bathroom and kneel down on the floor, perhaps leaning on the edge of the bath. • Wash your hands. • Place some clean towels, or clean clothing if you are in the car, between her knees. Have a clean towel, or other clean clothing, ready for wrapping the baby after it is born. • Gently receive the baby into your hands, and place it close to the mother. • Keep the baby warm, by wrapping it up or giving it to your partner to hold, and wrapping them both in a towel, blanket or what ever else is at hand. • Encourage her to sit and cuddle the baby, offering her breast for the baby to suckle. • Don't touch or cut the cord, leave it intact. • When the placenta appears, place it in a plastic container or bag and keep it close to the baby. The cord can be cut later by the midwife or ambulance paramedic. • Phone the hospital and either arrange for a midwife to visit, or take her to the hospital when she is ready, perhaps in the ambulance if it has arrived.
An induction is suggested to start labour	**Signs:** The pregnancy has extended beyond the expected date of birth. Signs of readiness for labour may be present. The baby may be showing signs of poor health. The mother may have an illness that cannot be treated properly while she is pregnant. **Possible reasons:** • If her body shows signs of being ready to start labour an induction may be suggested to "get her going", especially if the pregnancy has gone beyond a given date. • There may be no signs of any specific medical problem, but "social" reasons (e.g. imminent holidays) are suggested for starting the labour early. • Testing may have revealed that it would be better for the baby's health to be born early rather than waiting for labour to start naturally. • Effective treatment for a problem with the mother's health may not be possible until the baby is born. **Remedies:** Ask for the medical reason for the induction. You will find details about induction in *Preparing For Birth: Mothers.* Re-check the approximate birth day in consultation with the midwife. Try self-help strategies for starting the labour yourselves: • Sexual intercourse can trigger labour through stimulating your partner's hormones (oxytocin) and semen contains a hormone that assists the cervix to soften. Avoid having sex if the membranes have broken. • Castor oil (2 tablespoons in a glass of orange juice) encourages bowel movements which can also stimulate the uterus to start contracting. • Reflexology, acupressure and acupuncture can all be used to initiate labour. You will need to seek an appropriate therapist to help you with these remedies. If an induction is necessary, make sure she has a light meal first and encourage her to drink about a cupful of something nutritious (juice, tea etc) every hour throughout labour.

Trouble Shooting – Problems in labour CONTINUED

An induction is suggested to start labour (continued)	If the cervix is ready to dilate (ripe), rupturing the membranes (breaking the waters) may be all that is needed to start the contractions. If the cervix is not ready, a hormonal gel (Prostin) may be applied around the cervix. More details are contained in *Preparing For Birth: Mothers*. If these measures are not enough to start the uterus contracting naturally, a drip of oxytocin may be needed, and artificial oxytocin (Syntocinon) may be used to stimulate the uterus to contract. This is explained further in *Preparing For Birth: Mothers*. The contractions will be more painful, so use the ideas in this book to help her with this. There is no need for her to labour on the bed during an induction. She will be much more comfortable walking around, sitting on a chair or resting over pillows or a bean bag. Request a mobile drip stand so it can be wheeled about. 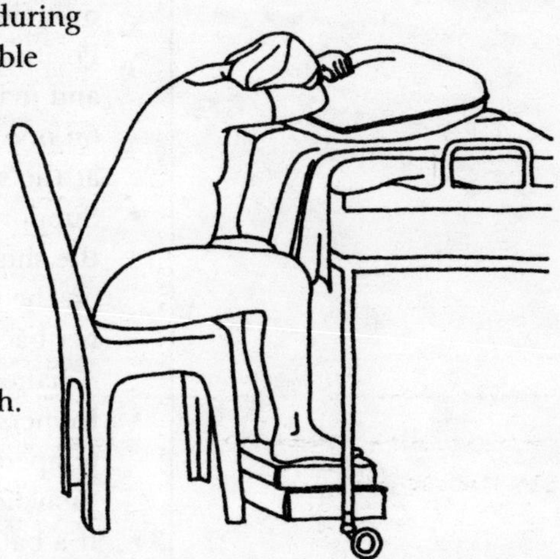 It is still possible to use the shower or bath following an induction. Once an induction is started, more frequent checks on the baby will be necessary and this may be easier with your partner in the shower rather than the bath. If an *electronic fetal monitor* is to be used, check the separate listing for ways of managing this comfortably.
She is experiencing a lot of pain during the labour	**Signs:** Some pain in labour is normal and healthy. However, she may have localised pain in one area, perhaps spreading further as the contraction continues. It may be felt mainly as a *backache* (see separate entry). **Possible reasons:** • As the cervix dilates, the stretching muscle tissues in the uterus signal what is happening by registering degrees of pain. This is necessary as a biofeedback mechanism to let your partner and her caregivers know how labour is progressing. • As the work required to open the cervix increases, especially towards the end of the first stage, the contractions become stronger and more painful. • Pain in one particular area may indicate a specific problem, such as a full bladder or an awkward position of the baby's head. **Remedies:** For the sake of the baby, it is best to try all the self-help strategies for easing labour pain before using pain-killing drugs, as these may have unwanted effects on the mother and baby. Make sure she is emptying her bladder every two hours. **Non-drug ways to ease the pain:** • Help her into a well supported, upright, forward-leaning position. This lessens the pressure on her back from the weight of the baby and makes it easier for the uterus to contract efficiently. Check in *Preparing For Birth: Mothers* for ideas. 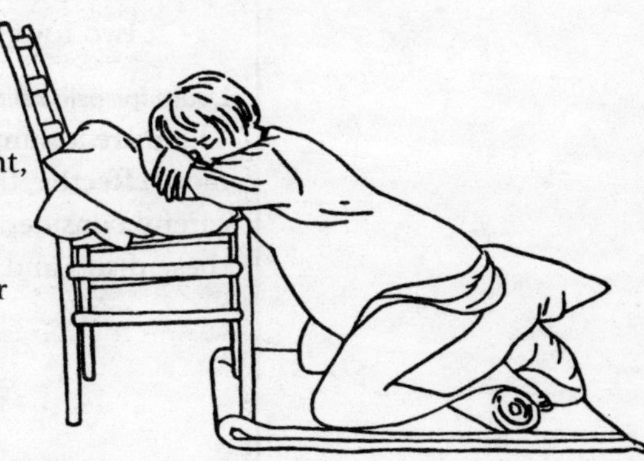 continued over

Trouble Shooting – Problems in labour CONTINUED

She is experiencing a lot of pain during the labour (continued)	• Verbal analgesia is often very effective. A few, well chosen words of support and understanding that are designed to acknowledge what she is doing and feeling may be all that is required. Midwives are skilled in offering encouraging, supportive words.
	• Walking, swaying and pelvic rocking can ease the pain and speed labour.
	• Hot packs, either the blue, jelly-filled variety, a heated wheat pack or hot, wet towels can be applied to sore spots for relief.
	• Massage is welcomed by many women in labour. Use a vegetable oil (even simple cooking oil can be used) to avoid friction, and rub slowly and rhythmically over the areas where is it hurting, usually her lower back. Position her in a well supported forward leaning position, and make sure you are comfortable too. Kneel on one knee and place the other leg at the side as shown.
	• Support her standing or sitting in the shower so that the water flows on the parts that are hurting, (usually her back, sometimes her lower tummy). A hand-held shower is useful to direct the water more easily.
	• Immersion in a bath or tub full of warm water can ease the pain. Keep the temperature below 37 degrees to avoid overheating her. Provide regular drinks to avoid dehydration and an inflatable pillow or folded towel for a head rest.
	• If a bath or shower are unavailable, an alternative source of heat and moisture are hot, wet towels. This is how they are used:
	  • You will need a bucket, three or four hand towels and a pair of rubber gloves to fit you and your support person.
	  • Fill the bucket with very hot water (perhaps topping it up from the tea kettle). The water will cool quickly once you start returning cold wet towels to the bucket.
	  • Place the bucket beside your partner. Put the hand towels in the bucket and put on the rubber gloves.
	  • When she gives a signal that a contraction is starting, lift a towel from the hot water, speedily wring it out as hard as possible so that there is no water dripping, unfold and drape over her lower back, or hold under her tummy if she prefers. Leave the towel in place until the start of the next contraction.
	  • With the next contraction, take off the cold towel and replace with a hot one. You will find a rhythm developing. If you have a helper, you could try two towels at a time, perhaps one on her back and another under her tummy.
	
	Drugs for pain relief:
	There are a number of drugs that may be offered for easing the pain, and some are more effective than others. All have side effects for the mother and the baby and need careful consideration before you decide to accept them. For detailed information on these drugs and their effects, see *Preparing For Birth: Mothers* manual.

Trouble Shooting – Problems in labour CONTINUED

Constant backache in labour	**Signs:** Continuous throbbing or dull aching in her lower back, becoming more intense during contractions. **Possible reasons:** • The baby is awkwardly positioned within the pelvis and its head is causing extra pressure on some of the bones and nerves in her lower back. • In second stage, pressure of the baby against the coccyx (tailbone) may cause intense pain if this bone has been damaged earlier in her life, perhaps in an accident. **Remedies:** Encourage the baby to turn into a more favourable alignment by positioning your partner in an "all fours" position over beanbags and pillows on a floormat. Rock her pelvis from side to side with your hands. Alternatively, encourage her to stand and swing her hips in big circles, to move the baby inside. Walk her up and down flights of stairs to enable pelvic tilting to move the baby. Apply steady, even pressure over her lower back, using your hands in the position shown. The application of combined water and heat may ease her pain. Try the bath (positioned on her knees, leaning forward over the end of the bath), the shower (kneeling on towels and leaning over a plastic chair or stool) or by applying hot, wet towels to her buttocks and lower back. Keep offering her regular drinks and snacks (if she wants them) as this labour is likely to be longer than expected. Encourage her to rest as much as possible to preserve her strength. Avoid giving her time limits or offering her interventions or drugs at first. Avoid having her *membranes ruptured artificially* as this removes the cushion of fluid around the baby that helps it to turn more easily. Take a break yourself from time to time, to conserve your energies. Try and have a short sleep yourself. Eat regularly, either nutritious snacks or a full meal. Arrange for additional help with the back rubbing – ask a friend of your partner's to come and help, or a close relative. The midwife may also be able to spend extra time while you take a break. Drugs may be offered, especially an epidural. Consider these carefully, especially the potential side effects for the mother and baby. For further information see *Preparing For Birth: Mothers* manual.

Trouble Shooting – Problems in labour CONTINUED

Labour progressing too slowly ("failure to progress")	**Signs:** Dilatation of the cervix is slower than 1 cm per hour, or has remained unchanged for some time. She may also be restless, anxious and in considerable pain during contractions. **Possible reasons:** • First labours are often much longer than subsequent labours. A slow, gradual build-up of contractions with little initial dilatation is quite normal in the absence of other signs or problems. • The baby is awkwardly positioned which is delaying its descent or restricting its ability to turn into a favourable position within the pelvis and trigger effective dilatation. • She is feeling anxious or pressured, causing her body to automatically slow labour until she feels safer and more secure. • The baby may be too big to fit through the pelvis (rare). **Remedies:** Increase her feelings of *security and safety*. Encourage her to take a bath or shower. Avoid giving her time limits (performance goals create additional stress). Keep offering her regular drinks, and if she desires, light snacks. Help her to change positions. Walk her around, perhaps up and down flights of stairs (but avoid over tiring her) Encourage her to rest, even doze between contractions. As long as the baby's heartbeat remains steady, offer her time for events to unfold naturally. *Artificially rupturing the membranes* will speed labour a little. Inserting a *drip of oxytocin* will speed labour artificially. A *Caesarean section* may be necessary if the baby is unable to fit through the pelvis. Try the remedies above as a means of clarifying this diagnosis.
Artificial rupture of the membranes is suggested	**Signs:** The staff want the labour to speed up. Uncertainty about possible fetal distress. A routine management procedure. **Possible reasons:** • Once the surrounding fluid has drained away, the baby will come into close contact with the cervix, which usually causes stronger contractions. This may increase the rate of dilatation of the cervix. See *augmentation*. • One way of checking for *fetal distress* is to observe the colour of the amniotic fluid. Rupturing the membranes is the easiest way to do this. • Doctors who prefer to actively manage labour usually include this procedure as part of this routine. **Remedies:** Labour can be speeded up by helping your partner into an upright position which will also bring the baby into closer contact with the cervix. The colour of the amniotic fluid can also be checked using an amnioscope to view the fluid through the cervix without breaking the membranes. Once the membranes are broken there is an increased risk of infection reaching the baby.

Trouble Shooting – Problems in labour CONTINUED

Artificial rupture of the membranes is suggested (continued)	To reduce this risk, request that further internal examinations be done only if there is a clear medical need for them. Removal of the cushioning fluid from around the baby can cause additional pressure from the stronger contractions on the baby, the cord and the placenta, and this may precipitate *fetal distress*.
Cramps or tingling ("pins and needles") in her legs, feet, or elsewhere	**Signs:** Her muscles cramp up with considerable pain and immobility. The nerves in her legs can be pinched from spending long periods without moving. **Possible reasons:** • The circulation system in pregnant women is naturally sluggish as a protective mechanism against the development of high blood pressure. • Look for sources of extra pressure: in the groin area, behind her knees, in her legs generally. **Remedies:** If the cramp is in her calf muscle, pull her toes up towards her knee as much as you can, stretching out the muscles until the cramp passes, then gently massage (using oil) over the area until the muscles feel soft. If the cramp is in her legs or feet, try to stretch out the muscles involved as much as you can, then when the spasm passes, massage over the affected area to improve the circulation. Encourage her to adopt another position less likely to result in cramps. If numbness develops, alter her position to relieve the pressure. Standing her up will enable her to easily move around, and reduce the risk of the problem recurring. Make sure her feet and legs are warm – long woolly socks are often welcome. The extra buoyancy from being in a bath will enable her to move freely and will assist in maintaining good circulation. If she chooses to squat in second stage, make sure that she stretches her legs in between each contraction by either standing up or by kneeling and leaning forward on a support.
She feels nauseous during labour	**Signs:** She tells you that she feels as though she will be sick. **Possible reasons:** • The condition may be due to her hormonal system. High levels of endorphins (the body's natural pain killing system) can create a side effect of nausea, especially towards the end of the first stage of labour. Nausea at this time is often a good sign of progress and doesn't last very long. **Remedies:** Sips of water, sucking on ice cubes or sweets, small drinks of non-acidic fruit juice may help her to feel better and reduce the risk of dehydration. Encourage her to vomit – once her stomach is empty she may feel better. Offer her a mouth rinse afterwards to get rid of the aftertaste. A common side effect of pethidine is nausea. Usually a second drug to counteract this will have been mixed with the pethidine before it is given. Check with the midwife. Sometimes the mask (nitrous oxide or entonox) can make a woman feel nauseated. Discontinuing its use may reduce the symptoms.

Trouble Shooting – Problems in labour CONTINUED

Your partner seems to be out of control	**Signs:** Wide eyes, restless and agitated behaviour, often accompanied by loud shouting, swearing, and calls for help and/or drugs. Vomiting and shaking may also be present. Often develops suddenly just when she has been managing the contractions well for some time. **Possible reason:** • Usually indicative of the transitional phase of labour, between first and second stages, especially if she was labouring comfortably earlier on. The uterus is changing its action from opening the cervix to pushing the baby out, causing new sensations which often feel very strange, overwhelming and difficult to manage. The contractions are also very close together, with little recovery time in between. **Remedies:** If you are unsure what is happening, ask the midwife to evaluate the situation and provide feedback and support for you both. Remind your partner that these feelings are excellent indicators of progress. Tell her that she is in the transitional phase of labour. Try to stay calm yourself. Ignore the irrational behaviour and try to ease the symptoms until this phase passes – usually half to one hour is all that is needed. Discourage her from accepting drugs. By the time an epidural is administered, this phase may be over, and she will then have difficulty pushing the baby out herself. Pethidine given at this point can cause breathing and sucking difficulties for the baby after birth. The mask (nitrous oxide/entonox) may help reduce the pain for a few contractions, but avoid extended use as its effects on the baby are unknown. Help her to change positions and make her as comfortable as you can. Offer the bath or a shower as these are very effective ways of easing the pain at this time. If she is unwilling to move to the bathroom, use hot, wet towels on her buttocks, lower back or tummy to ease the pain. Create feelings of privacy, *security and safety*. Have a bowl ready in case she needs to vomit. Remind yourself that this phase will pass and she will return to more normal behaviours once second stage begins.
She is becoming dehydrated	**Signs:** Dry mouth and lips. Lack of energy, acute fatigue. Slowing of the labour. **Possible reasons:** • Labour began some time after the last meal, with few snacks eaten since. • Inappropriate restrictions on food and drinks imposed by hospital staff. • Not enough fluids have been offered: approximately one cup of fluid per hour should be offered. • Long periods of time spent in the bath without adequate fluids to drink. **Remedies:** Make sure she has a light snack when labour is beginning, and sips drinks frequently throughout the labour. A flexible straw often makes this easier.

Trouble Shooting – Problems in labour CONTINUED

She is becoming dehydrated (continued)	Take your own snacks and drinks with you to the hospital, to be sure you have something appropriate available. There is evidence that restricting food and fluids in labour leads to higher Caesarean section rates due to the uterus running out of energy and the contractions stalling as a result *(failure to progress)*. Make sure she continues to have regular drinks if she is spending time in the shower or bath. She will not absorb much water from her surroundings, and the steamy atmosphere can make her sweat more, leading to dehydration. If the dehydration is severe, a drip may be inserted by the midwife to increase her fluid intake.
You are feeling faint at the thought (or sight) of blood	**Signs:** Feeling faint and dizzy, even nauseous. **Possible reasons:** • A previous life experience may have affected you. **Remedies:** One advantage of labour taking time is that you have a chance to get used to the sights and smells associated with birth. Keep busy and involved. Having a job to do puts the focus onto your partner's needs, rather than your own reactions. If you do feel faint, go outside and get a breath of fresh air. Make sure you take regular breaks and remember to eat – when you are tired and hungry you may be more emotionally vulnerable. Most fathers, even the most fearful, are surprised at how they are drawn into the birth process, finding it exciting and emotionally uplifting. Many forget their own reactions completely and discover hidden strengths and abilities which can be a revelation in itself.
You are in a panic	**Signs:** Feelings of being "out of control", helpless and frightened. Restlessness and agitation. Shouting, demanding action and assistance, wanting to pass on responsibility to others. **Possible reasons:** • You may feel unable to help, be anxious about what is happening, or be frightened that your partner or the baby is in danger. • The first time you witness a birth can be very scary, and the hospital setting can feel intimidating. • Your partner may seem to be a "different person" when she is in labour and react in ways you have never seen before. This can be quite upsetting. **Remedies:** Try and find out about labour and birth in advance so you have some idea of what is going on. Visit the hospital and meet her care givers before the big event. Consult the midwife if you are unsure about anything – they are there to help. Consider taking an extra support person to help you share the responsibility for making her comfortable. Your partner may be able to suggest someone, such as a close friend, her sister, mother or other relative. continued over

Trouble Shooting – Problems in labour CONTINUED

You are in a panic. (continued)	Take regular breaks for food and rest during the labour. When you are tired you can easily become more emotional than normal. If you feel panic setting in, get help. Talk to the midwife who can explain what is happening and help you share the responsibility for assisting your partner. Leave the room and have a change of scene. Make sure there is someone else to support your partner while you are away.
The labour has started naturally, but speeding it up (augmentation) using a drip is suggested	**Signs:** Although contractions may be present, they may not be very strong or dilating the cervix. **Possible reasons:** • The labour may be starting slowly, and be quite normal. • There may be other reasons why the contractions are not very effective – see *labour too slow*. • The staff may want the baby to be born by a given time. **Remedies:** Ask if there is a medical problem (the midwife can tell if your partner and the baby are both in good health). If there isn't one, consider the suggestions listed under *labour progressing slowly*. If the baby or your partner has a medical problem, consider the treatments that have been suggested, and take time to decide what to do. If you decide to have the membranes ruptured in an effort to speed up labour, be aware that the following few contractions will be much stronger than before. Help her to prepare for this by assisting her into an upright position so she can move around. See *induction* for more ideas. 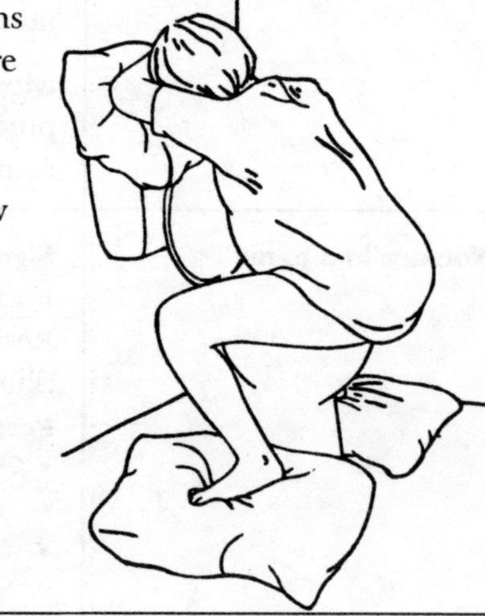 With each subsequent contraction there will be a flow of amniotic fluid, so make sure she has panties on and thick pads in place to catch the trickles. She may prefer to sit on the toilet or a bedpan for a while until the flow settles down. Once the membranes have broken (naturally or artificially) anything that enters her vagina could cause infection, and internal examinations should be carried out only if absolutely necessary.
The membranes break and the amniotic fluid (waters) is a yellow/brown/green colour	**Signs:** The fluid is not clear, but coloured. It can vary from pale yellow to thick, dark green/brown. **Possible reasons:** • The baby may be overdue. Moving the bowels (practising!) can be a sign that the baby is ready to be born. • Sometimes the baby opens its bowels because it is distressed. The colour of the fluid is important: a pale colour suggests that this may have happened some hours or days ago. If the fluid is darker, and particularly if it is sticky and thick, then the baby may be distressed now. **Remedies:** The midwife will check the baby's condition, using a fetal stethoscope to listen to its heartbeat or an *electronic fetal monitor*.

Trouble Shooting – Problems in labour CONTINUED

The membranes break and the amniotic fluid (waters) is a yellow/brown/green colour (continued)	If there does not appear to be problem at the present time, continue to support your partner as before. A doctor may be called to advise on the baby's condition. A *Caesarean section* may be suggested if immediate rescue of the baby is necessary, especially in the first stage of labour. In second stage, forceps or vacuum may be used instead to speed up the birth.
The baby is showing signs of fetal distress	**Signs:** The baby's heartbeat is dropping very low, especially after contractions. The *amniotic fluid may be coloured*. **Possible reasons:** • The baby may be pressing on the umbilical cord or the cord may be compressed between the baby and the wall of the uterus. These problems can occur following the *rupture of the membranes* when the cushioning fluid escapes or due to the position adopted by the mother during labour. • If the labour has been long the baby may become fatigued. • If the contractions are long, strong and closely spaced, the baby may become distressed by a lack of oxygen. This is more likely to occur with an *induction* or *augmentation*. • If drugs have been used during labour, these may affect the baby over time. • If an *electronic fetal monitor* is being used, the belts may be poorly placed or have slipped out of position, resulting in a faulty recording. • Prolonged pushing and breath holding in second stage (especially if the mother is *lying on her back* or semi sitting) may reduce the oxygen supply to the baby and cause fetal distress. **Remedies:** Ask the midwife to carefully assess the situation. A doctor will probably be called to advise so talk to them both to get a clear idea of the situation. Your partner will be aware that her caregivers are concerned about the baby and this will increase her anxiety, which is turn can slow labour and make it more painful. Including her in the discussions may help reduce her anxiety. While the situation is being assessed, there are many things you can do to assist her: Try changing your partner's position. Encourage her to sit, either leaning forward over pillows or the back of a chair or against you. Discourage her from lying down on her back for any procedure, as the weight of the baby will interfere with her circulation and that, in turn, can reduce the oxygen flow to the baby. Checking the baby's heartbeat, internal and external examinations and *electronic fetal monitoring* can all be done with the woman sitting or standing up. Avoid having the *membranes ruptured artificially*. If there is a drip running to stimulate contractions, ask the midwife to reduce the flow of the drug, to slow the frequency of the contractions. This will give the baby more time to recover between contractions. If the labour is being induced, it may be possible to discontinue the drip altogether once the contractions have become established so a less stressful and more natural pattern of contractions can develop. Allow time for the baby to adapt to the changes you have made. Ask the midwife to check the baby frequently using a regular fetal stethoscope instead

continued over

	of a sonicaid or hand held doppler. The baby may react to the ultrasound used in this equipment by moving more and as a result be harder to locate. If fetal distress is suspected, an *electronic fetal monitor* with an scalp electrode attached to the baby's head will give a more accurate and continuous measure of the baby's well being. If an *electronic fetal monitor* is used, check that the external belts are accurately placed and properly recording. If a scalp electrode is attached to the baby's head, it can become less reliable during second stage if it is accidentally pressed against the vagina during the birth. Seek a second opinion, especially regarding the interpretation of an electronic trace, as these are notoriously difficult to read. Try to stay calm and think clearly. If the condition persists, a *Caesarean section* may become necessary.
An electronic fetal monitor is suggested	**Signs:** A routine part of the hospital's or caregiver's approach to managing birth. The baby's heart rate may need closely monitoring following another procedure, such as rupturing the membranes, an *induction*, or once drugs have been given for pain relief. Further information can be found in *Preparing For Birth: Mothers*. **Possible reasons:** • Although there is no scientific evidence that their use improves birth outcomes for normal healthy mothers and babies, the use of an electronic fetal monitor is often presented as a routine procedure. • If the baby is reacting poorly to interventions in labour an electronic fetal monitor gives continuous information about the baby's well being. **Remedies:** Request that the midwife uses her fetal stethoscope to listen to the baby. Her readings can be just as accurate as the machine. Suggest that the monitor be used periodically, for say 10 minutes every hour, and that it be removed in between. This will only possible if external equipment is used. It is not necessary or advisable for your partner to lie down while attached to an electronic fetal monitor. An upright position, either sitting, standing or kneeling improves the blood flow and therefore oxygen supply to the baby. Your partner's movements will be limited by the length of the monitor's cables. If available, a battery operated personal telemetry unit that beams the readings to a central monitoring station will enable your partner to move about freely. If she is moving about with external belts attached, make sure they stay in position. You may need to hold them to ensure continuous recordings are being made. If the printed trace shows gaps, ask the midwife to check the equipment, as it may have slipped or be faulty. Some women find the sounds of the heartbeat comforting and others find it distracting. Adjust the monitor's sound level accordingly. Try not to make the machinery the centre of attention. Remember that it is your partner having the baby, not the electronic equipment, and give her your attention at all times.

Trouble Shooting – Problems in labour CONTINUED

The baby is not moving down through the pelvis	**Signs:**

Signs:
Despite strong, and often very painful contractions over some hours, the baby does not appear to be moving lower into the pelvis.

Possible reasons:

- The position of the baby's head may be making it difficult for the baby to turn into a more favourable position.
- There may be a big bag of waters in front of the baby's head, cushioning its descent.
- Her bladder may be full, delaying the descent of the baby.
- The baby may be too big to fit through the pelvis (rare).

Remedies:
Confirm the nature of the problem with the midwife. Her regular checks to assess progress will help reveal the situation.

If the baby is awkwardly positioned, help your partner to try various positions, to ease her pain and encourage the baby to turn. Alternating with walking around may help.

Pelvic rocking, either from walking up stairs, swinging the hips in large circles or tilting while on hands and knees may help the baby to rotate.

Try pressing on her sacro-iliac joints (the midwife an help you locate these joints on her lower back) while she is kneeling and leaning right over a bean bag or pillows. This puts pressure on the pubic joint and encourages it to spread a little, making more space for the baby to move down into the pelvis. If this pressure causes pain in the pubic area, then discontinue.

If progress is being delayed by a large bag of amniotic fluid in front of the baby's head, rupturing the membranes may speed progress. Alternatively, she may decide to wait until the membranes break naturally to ensure the baby is well protected in the mean time. If the baby is otherwise well positioned and not too large, progress may be rapid once the membranes break.

Encourage her to empty her bladder. Sitting on the toilet may help, but a bedpan may be more convenient.

She needs to empty her bladder every two hours during labour (at least). If she is unsuccessful, the midwife may offer to insert a catheter into her bladder to release the urine and make more space.

In second stage, deep squatting will open up the pelvis to enable the baby to move down further. Support her fully as she squats or provide something solid for her to hold onto for balance. Encourage her to stand up between contractions to avoid restricting her circulation, which can give her *cramps* in the legs.

If the baby is still high in the pelvis when the cervix is fully open and still shows no sign of moving down, a *Caesarean section* will probably be necessary.

If she has been pushing in second stage and the baby has moved part of the way, forceps or vacuum (ventouse) may be used to turn the baby so it can be born through the vagina. If this fails, then a *Caesarean section* will be necessary.

Bleeding during labour	**Signs:** Fresh, bright blood escaping from the vagina. **Possible reason:** • This is a rare condition. • The placenta has begun to separate from the uterus before the baby has been born. This is a very rare condition, and the reason why it has happening is unlikely to be clear. **Remedy:** This is an emergency situation. If you are at home, call an ambulance and get her to the hospital as fast as you can. If you are in the hospital, alert the midwife immediately. A *Caesarean section* is the most likely outcome.
She is asked to lie on her back to give birth	**Signs:** The baby is about to be born and the midwife or doctor requests that she lie down on her back. **Possible reasons:** • Habit – most care givers were trained to assist at births with the woman lying on her back. • Inexperience with assisting women give birth in upright positions. • Your partner has been labouring on the bed and a recumbent position is adopted automatically. • She is unable to adopt a more natural position because the drugs she has been given for pain make it difficult for her to move. **Remedies:** If your partner has been labouring in an upright position, especially at the end of the first stage, encourage her to remain like this for the birth. You may have to physically hold her to increase her comfort and stability as she pushes the baby out. Keep her off the bed during labour. She will be more comfortable if she has a floor mat to stand or kneel on. Request that the midwife assists, especially if the doctor is unwilling or unable to help. If she has little movement in her legs due to an epidural anaesthetic, wait until the anaesthetic wears off. She will then be able to move into a better position. If she is feeling dizzy due to pethidine, give her good physical support to increase her feeling of security when she is upright. You may need a second person to help you. Don't rush her as she gives birth. She will have an automatic urge to push and her body will tell her how much effort is needed. Gravity will encourage the baby to move down through her vagina. An episiotomy is rarely needed. Allowing time for the tissues to stretch will reduce the risk of tearing, and an upright position enables the vagina to open naturally. Encourage her to keep her eyes closed and to ignore any instructions about pushing being given by care givers. It is best for her to use her own instincts as she gives birth, to reduce trauma to the baby and to protect her own body.

Trouble Shooting – Problems in labour CONTINUED

A complication has occurred and a Caesarean section is recommended	**Signs:** The baby is showing signs of acute *fetal distress*: its heartbeat is slowing and the amniotic fluid is stained dark. The labour is progressing very slowly, or not at all. Your partner is bleeding during the labour. The umbilical cord has fallen through the cervix into the vagina and is in front of the baby's head. The baby is poorly positioned or very large and is not moving down through the pelvis. **Possible reasons:** • There are many reasons why a Caesarean section may be suggested. For a full list, see *Preparing For Birth: Mothers* manual. Approximately 10–15% of all babies will need a Caesarean birth. • Complications may have developed as a result of earlier interventions (e.g. the induction has failed to produce adequate progress). • The *induction* or *augmentation* may have failed to get the baby born within a given period of time. • The drugs that have been used to stimulate the labour may be affecting the baby. • The drugs used for pain may be causing distress to the baby. • Unexpected complications can occur, such as sudden bleeding or the prolapse of the umbilical cord that can be life threatening for the unborn baby. • The baby may remain in an awkward position that makes a vaginal birth impossible. **Remedies:** Ask for details of the problem and discuss the situation with your partner. This may be an emergency situation that is best handled by the hospital staff and the doctor. If there is no medical emergency, ask about alternative approaches with the midwife. Try and stay calm. More than anything, your partner needs strong support from you and the midwife. If there is enough time, your partner will be given an epidural anaesthetic (if one is not already in place) or a spinal anaesthetic. Try and make her as comfortable as you can while this is being done. You can request to be present during the Caesarean, if you wish. You will be dressed for the operating theatre in a gown, mask, gloves, booties and a paper hat. The procedure for a Caesarean birth is described in *Preparing For Birth: Mothers*. If the baby is well enough, it will be given to you to hold after the birth. Try to help your partner see and hold the baby too – if you assist, it should also be possible to put the baby to her breast. If an emergency Caesarean is necessary, she will be given a general anaesthetic. You may still be able to attend the birth, however, if there is not time to dress you for the theatre you may have to wait in the recovery area instead. If the baby is taken to the intensive care nursery, stay with the baby so that you know what is happening and can report back to your partner. She will be anxious to know about the baby's condition, and if you are in the nursery you can see what is being done for your child.

Trouble Shooting – Problems after the birth

Bleeding immediately after the birth (post-partum haemorrhage)	**Signs:** A sudden gush of bright red blood just after the baby is born. **Possible reasons:** • The uterus is not contracting tightly around the placenta as it separates from the uterus, allowing blood to escape rapidly. **Remedies:** This is an emergency and the midwife or doctor will act quickly to stop the bleeding. Your partner will be given an injection to make the uterus contract strongly and the placenta will be removed as quickly as possible. Help your partner to put the baby to her breast as this will also encourage the uterus to contract.
Bleeding some time after the birth	**Signs:** A flow of bright red blood in the days after the birth. **Possible reasons:** • There is always a flow of blood (similar to a heavy period) in the days after birth, as the uterus shrinks back to its normal size and the placental site heals. • If there is sudden bleeding, especially with small or large clots of blood, it is likely that some small fragments of placenta or membranes which did not come away just after the birth are being expelled from her uterus now. She may also experience some cramping when this occurs. **Remedies:** Telephone the hospital if you need more information or guidance. Once the clots have been passed, the bleeding usually stops. If it persists, take your partner to the hospital to be checked by the midwife and a doctor. Stay calm. Keep her warm and quiet. If the bleeding continues it may be necessary for a doctor to perform a D & C (dilatation and curettage) to remove any remaining fragments of placenta. This will be done in the hospital under general anaesthetic.
Your partner is having problems breastfeeding the baby	**Signs:** There are a number of different problems that can occur with breastfeeding such as: cracked, sore nipples, engorged, swollen breasts fussy, unsettled baby baby losing weight or gaining weight very slowly. **Possible reasons:** • The most common cause of breastfeeding problems is poor attachment of the baby to the breast. • Restricted feed times may be a contributing factor. • A breast infection may be involved. **Remedies:** Get help from a knowledgeable midwife, a breastfeeding counsellor or a Lactation Consultant, by phoning the hospital, going to the local baby health clinic, contacting a breastfeeding support group or checking the phone book. Your local book shop or lending library may have useful reference books as well. Offer your partner encouragement and support at this time. Your understanding will go a long way to enabling her to enjoy breastfeeding and getting it right.

Trouble Shooting – Problems after the birth CONTINUED

The baby is in the intensive care unit	**Signs:** The baby is taken to the special care or intensive care nursery for observation or treatment following the birth. **Possible reasons:** • The baby has a problem that needs treatment. • The birth was complicated and the baby may need close observation for a period of time. • Some hospitals still have a policy that following either a Caesarean or forceps birth, babies are routinely observed in the special care nursery for a set period of time. **Remedies:** Having a baby in an intensive care unit or special care nursery is a traumatic experience. You will both need emotional support and possibly counselling to help you come to terms with the situation. Working through this together will make it easier to adjust to the circumstances. Ask questions about the treatments being given. It helps to know what is being done for your baby. Enquire about community groups that offer additional support. These groups are often a good source of practical information about caring for the baby in hospital and at home. It is still possible to breastfeed, and breast milk will be best nourishment for your child. Obtain a breast pump if necessary (hospital staff can advise where they can be hired) and encourage your partner as she establishes her milk supply.
Your notes:	

At the end of the day

After the baby has been born, you will probably be feeling a whole array of emotions: elation, exhaustion, amazement, anxiety, fulfilment, confusion . . . .

Whatever you are feeling it will be quite normal, and it may take some time for you to come to terms with your emotions at this point. Talking about the events and your reactions with your partner, other fathers, or caregivers may help. It is important not to bottle up these feelings, but to acknowledge them and express them as spontaneously as you can. Your whole world has changed, and it is expected that you will react in your own way to this momentous event.

Your journey as a father is only just beginning, and unimaginable pleasures (and some pain) await you.

You will never be the same person again, and this change in your circumstances will give you enormous opportunities for self development and discovery, as you create new relationships that will add richness and depth to your life. It is a very special time and a unique experience that only you can have. Take what life has given you and enjoy it to the full.

COMMUNITY RESOURCES

There is lots of help available for new families in your community. The Government provides a range of professional services and there are community groups that offer support and information especially for parents with particular needs. You may care to complete this list with the help of your childbirth educator, who will have phone numbers and names for your local area. The telephone book and community information services may also provide useful contacts.

BREASTFEEDING SUPPORT AND INFORMATION

Community groups

Ph

Lactation Consultant

Ph

Well Baby Clinic (Baby Health Centre, Health Visitor etc)

Ph

New mothers groups

Ph

General Practitioner

Ph

Paediatrician

Ph

Post-natal depression

Ph

Mothercraft services (Tresillian, Plunket, etc)

Ph

Counselling services (Telephone hotlines etc, social worker etc)

Ph

Cot death support

Ph

Stillbirth and neonatal death

Ph